Understanding Body Stress Release

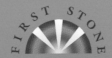

Contents

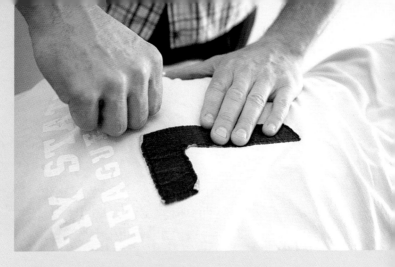

1

What Is
Body Stress Release?

Body Stress Release, or BSR, is a unique complementary health technique that assists the body in restoring its in-built ability to heal and maintain itself.

Body Stress Release was pioneered by South Africans, Gail and Ewald Meggersee, in the early 1980s. Most BSR practitioners are located in South Africa and the UK, although Holland, Germany, Iceland, Namibia, Australia, New Zealand and the USA also have them.

In everyday life we are subjected to various kinds of stress. There is mechanical

Clients are amazed that a gentle technique can be so effective

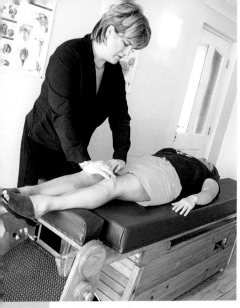

BSR is carried out with the client fully-clothed.

stress, such as falls, accidents, heavy lifting and incorrect posture. Chemical stress may occur in the form of air pollutants, additives and colorants in food, as well as harmful chemicals in some cosmetics and cleaning products. Furthermore, we all experience mental and emotional stress.

When these stresses accumulate to the point of stress overload, the body is unable to adapt to them and tension becomes stored in physical structures – this is termed body stress. It may cause pain, stiffness, numbness or postural distortion. The resulting nerve compression disturbs the body's communication system and undermines its normal functioning.

While the person is lying fully-clothed on a uniquely designed couch, the BSR practitioner does a series of pressure tests, activating the neuro-muscular reflexes of the body. In this way the body is used as a bio-feedback mechanism and its responses indicate the exact sites of locked-in stress. The practitioner then applies light but definite pressure in the precise directions indicated. This enables the body to release the body stress, thereby restoring communication and its self-healing ability.

People often ask what BSR is like, and whether it compares to any other technique that they may have tried. To understand Body Stress Release, it needs to be experienced. It is completely unique. It does not involve massage, manipulation, the use of any machines, or medication.

Clients are amazed that such a gentle technique can be so effective.

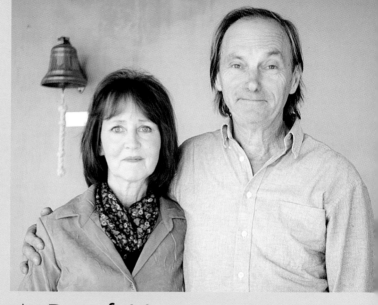

2 A Brief History

Body Stress Release was developed by South Africans Ewald and Gail Meggersee in the early 1980s, in response to Ewald's own crippling adversity.

After falling from a tree at the age of five, Ewald experienced continuous pain in his lower back and shooting pains in his legs. His school days were unbearable; because of intense pain he couldn't sit still at a desk and was shouted at for fidgeting. He would often collapse from a deep ache in his knees if asked to stand for any period of time. At 15, he was told that his pain and severe cramping were psychosomatic because no one could find any physical cause for his problems.

Ewald qualified as an industrial chemist and met and married Gail, a teacher. His pain did not ease. He would scream out in his sleep and leap out of bed in the grip of intense cramping in his calf muscles. On occasions he would wake up feeling no sensation from the waist down, and he would be forced to roll out of bed onto the floor, pulling himself up via the wardrobe for support while he waited for sensation to return to his legs.

Ewald's nightmare became a regular occurrence. He feared going to sleep at night, not knowing if he was going to wake up permanently paralysed. It became so bad that he faced losing his job and spending the rest of his life in a wheelchair.

Over the years Ewald had received temporary relief from regular chiropractic adjustments, but the pain would always return. He and Gail felt they had nothing to lose by going to America to train as chiropractors. They hoped to discover something that had been missed, and to find a way to identify the source of Ewald's pain and reverse his worsening condition.

> *He feared going to sleep at night, not knowing if he was going to wake up permanently paralysed.*

During their studies in America, they met a retired chiropractor, Dr Richard van Rumpt, who had researched an approach completely different to chiropractic manipulation. He talked about listening to the body and using it as a bio-feedback mechanism. When the Meggersees returned to South Africa, they built on his method of reading the body's responses.

They began working together on clients and this enabled them to discover how the body automatically reacts to stress in a highly organised way. The stored stress occurs as lines of tension in specific directions. They also discovered how the sites of body stress are inter-connected. This research led to the creation of the technique named Body Stress Release.

POPULARITY GROWTH

Although still relatively new in the UK and Europe, tens of thousands of South Africans have benefited from Body Stress Release since the Meggersees opened their original practice in Cape Town, in 1981.

Many of their clients, like Ewald himself, had tried traditional avenues of medical

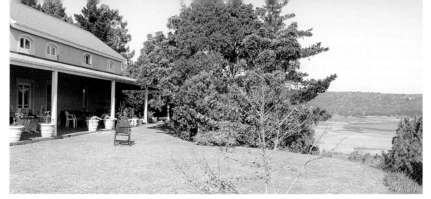

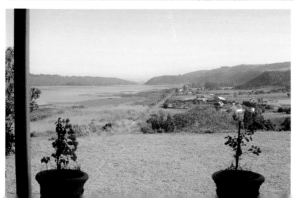

Above: The Body Stress Release Academy in South Africa.
Left: The view from the Academy.

treatment, without success. But now the couple had found a gentle, almost miraculous way of enhancing the body's own healing powers by releasing long-held stress in the body.

They knew it worked because their prime guinea pig, Ewald, had gone from being a near cripple to regaining his strength. Ewald regained a pain-free body, which he now describes as 'being as fit as a teenager's'. Today, at 62, Ewald reports that his body continues to upgrade with regular BSR.

THE BSR ACADEMY, SOUTH AFRICA

In 1997, the Meggersees moved to Rondevlei on South Africa's Garden Route, where they relocated the Body Stress Release Academy. The growth of Body Stress Release continues worldwide, albeit slowly, as the Meggersees are the only teachers of the technique.

The BSR practitioner-training course is an intensive, five-month programme. Twenty-four students are trained during each year.

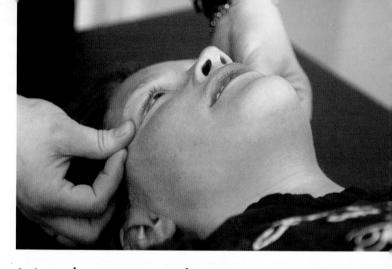

Understanding
Body Stress

The dictionary defines stress as 'a force, pressure, tension or constraining influence'.

Not all stress is harmful. We require a certain level of stress to promote growth and development, through repeated positive adaptations. Without stress we would be unable to survive. When we are frightened, our 'fight or flight' response comes into action.

WHAT CAUSES BODY STRESS?
Stress becomes a negative factor only when it goes beyond our ability to adapt to it. When stress gets too much to handle, it reaches the level of overload and becomes stored in the body as 'body stress'. As a result, the body is less able to deal with any further stress that it is subjected to and it enters a cycle of negative adaptation.

Body stress occurs instantly – the moment the point of stress overload is reached. Of course, every individual has a different threshold of stress overload but the effects are the same. Overload triggers the body's survival mode of action. This is automatically activated by a reflex reaction, which is controlled by mechanisms located in the spinal cord. This action does not involve the brain and may occur anywhere in the body. The tissues surrounding the site of involvement tighten in order to protect the area. It is very noticeable how the overlying muscles contract in order to restrict movement.

As muscles are designed to move and support the body structures, they cross over the joints. When body stress occurs, muscles tighten to restrict movement and the involved joints become squeezed together. This compressive force has an impact on the nerves. When it occurs in the spine, the pressure on the spinal nerves has a far-reaching, highly disruptive effect on the body's communication system.

The brain may not be aware of the site of body stress, so the body's self-healing mechanisms are not activated to release the stored tension. The body enters a situation where it requires some outside assistance to release the stress, and this is the function of the BSR practitioner.

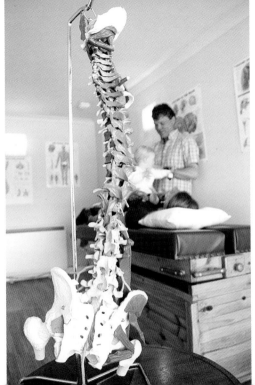

Pressure on the spinal nerves when body stress occurs in the spine has a far-reaching, disruptive effect on the body's communication system. The body then requires some outside assistance, and this is the function of the BSR practitioner.

17

RELEASING BODY STRESS

If locked-in stress is not released, over a period of time the overlying muscles in the area will undergo increased contraction. The pressure on the nerves will disturb the communication of the body. This may lead to:

- Aches and pains or numbness
- Loss of flexibility, leading to postural distortion
- Loss of efficiency in the body's functioning
- Illness
- Degeneration.

When stress becomes locked into the body, it becomes necessary for it to be released by means of outside help, such as the Body Stress Release technique, or it will cause ongoing problems.

CAUSES AND EFFECTS OF BODY STRESS

There are three types of stress that may affect the body: mechanical stress, mental/emotional stress, and chemical stress.

They impact the body in many different ways.

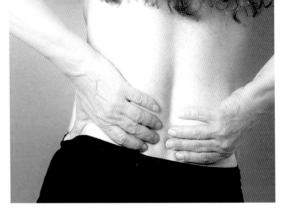

The jarring effects of accidents and falls may cause body stress to become locked into the lower back.

The lower back

The jarring effect of accidents and falls may cause body stress to become locked into the lower back. Also, heavy or incorrect lifting or bending may strain ligaments and muscles and result in stress becoming stored in the body. The wrong kind of exercises, such as those that involve twisting movements or repeated forward bending, may stress the lower spine.

Another cause is poor

19

posture, especially sitting in a slumped position, which reverses the normal lumbar curve. Sitting slumped may give temporary relief from back pain, as it causes the joint spaces to open up at the back and thus reduce pressure on the discs, but over time the back walls of the discs may weaken and develop a bulge. This would result in pressure being exerted on a spinal nerve.

Irritation to the spinal nerves of the lower back may result in back pain, and this can be referred along the nerve pathways into the abdomen, groin, hips, legs or feet. Often, pain is felt along the large sciatic nerve, which passes through the buttock and down the back of the leg. There may also be a sensation of numbness in any of these areas. Muscle function may be affected, resulting in stiffness or weakness. The compression effect in the lower back may be so severe that the back muscles lock up in a protective spasm, pulling the spine sideways or forwards.

While body stress remains stored in the lower back, the

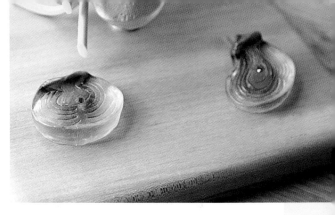

Over time, poor posture may cause the back walls of the intervertebral discs to weaken and develop a bulge. This results in pressure being exerted on the spinal nerve.

irritation to the nerves may undermine or disturb the normal functioning of the areas and the organs they supply. Thus body stress may lead to digestive problems (such as constipation or diarrhoea), bladder complaints, and may adversely affect sexual function.

Sometimes, a person may not be aware of body stress in the lower back, other than feeling stiffness on arising in the morning. After BSR, a person

21

may be pain-free for a period and then experience a return of the problem for no apparent reason. This signals that the lower back is ready to undergo a further, deeper release of body stress.

If body stress has been present in the lower back for a long time (the cause may have originated in childhood), it may be necessary for the stored tension to be released in layers over a period of time.

As the foundation of the spine, the lower back area affects the stability of the rest of the spine.

Therefore, if body stress is stored in the lumbar area, muscular tension will be referred to the upper back and neck.

The mid and upper back

Mechanical stress caused by working in a hunched or twisted posture may strain the chest and back areas. Lifting heavy objects, or holding something up for a long time, may cause problems. Body stress may also occur as a result of a painful spasm of the diaphragm.

Other reasons for body stress in this area may be emotional

tension, such as shock or anxiety.

Other causes may include chemical factors, such as irritation from eating or drinking something spicy, acidic or very cold. Body stress in the diaphragm muscle may result in indigestion or heartburn, or a feeling of breathlessness.

In addition, if there is body stress in the lower back, it may be referred into the muscles of the chest and upper back.

The effects felt can include a mild, nagging ache in the upper back between the shoulder blades, or possibly a persistent itch. Body stress may also manifest as a severe stabbing pain in this area, or in the chest. The pain is worsened by deep breathing.

Body stress in the mid and upper back may have an impact on the nerve supply to the various internal organs, such as the heart, lungs, kidney and bladder, and may interfere with normal function.

The neck
There are various factors that may cause body stress in the neck area:

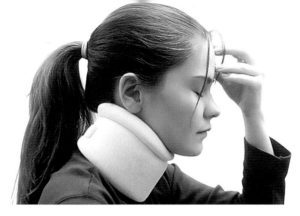

Many factors can cause body stress in the neck, including whiplash.

- Mechanical causes: Jarring or jerking the neck, as in a fall or whiplash in a car accident; working or reading with the head tilted downwards for lengthy periods; twisting the neck, as in reversing a car.

- Mental/emotional causes: Emotions such as intense anger, anxiety or shock can cause a person to hunch the shoulders and tighten the neck muscles. A state of ongoing depression will also bring about postural distortion. In addition, the physical discomfort resulting from body stress will reinforce the negative emotions, creating a vicious circle.

- Chemical causes: Exposure to harmful chemicals may severely irritate the nervous system and cause the neck muscles to tighten, e.g. chemicals may be inhaled, such as car fumes and insecticides; substances may be absorbed through the skin, such as cleaning materials and certain cosmetics. Some people react adversely to certain foods and to preservatives and additives. Very often, an infection (such as the flu or cold virus) may also result in neck stress.

Body stress stored in the neck may cause pain and stiffness and an inability to fully turn the head.

As the lower neck supplies the nerves to the arms, there may be pain or numbness in the shoulder, arm or hand. Muscles may be weakened, resulting in difficulty grasping objects.

Tension in the neck may cause

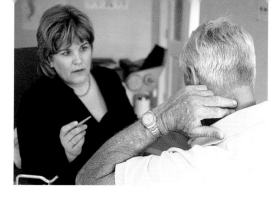

Body stress stored in the neck may cause pain and stiffness and an inability to fully turn the head.

headaches or pain in the face or jaw. There may be a sensation of dizziness or nausea. The pressure may irritate the nerve pathways that connect with the eyes, nose and mouth, and this could adversely affect vision and the senses of smell and taste.

Another effect may be a burning, dry mouth or excess saliva.

Body stress in the neck area may also have an impact on the nerve connections to the internal organs, such as the heart, lungs and digestive system, undermining normal function.

The shoulder

The upper arm bone fits into a shallow socket on the side of the shoulder blade. As this allows a wide range of movement, the shoulder joint is easily subjected to body stress. Reaching above the head, stretching the arm backwards, jarring effects in sports like tennis, may put strain on the ligaments and muscles of the shoulder, resulting in tension becoming locked into the joint.

The shoulder may be stiff and painful. If there is a build up of inflammation, the pain may be intense. Most likely the release of this stored tension would have to be carried out over a period of time, to enable the joint to stabilise and healing to take place.

In a long-term case of body stress of the shoulder, the joint may become 'frozen'. In certain such cases, full movement of the shoulder is restored immediately after the stress is released. In other cases, this may occur only after several sessions of BSR. Therefore, to avoid the problem progressing to the stage of immobility, it is

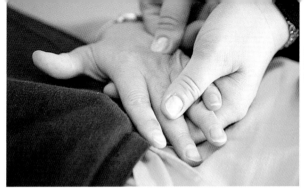

Body stress being released from the hand.

advisable to have the shoulder attended to as soon as possible after an injury occurs.

The elbow, wrist and hand
These joints may be stressed by jarring the arm, as in a fall, by twisting movements (such as using a screwdriver or opening a tight jar), or by vigorous actions such as using woodworking tools.

Tension becomes locked into the elbow joint, between the small wrist bones or between the hand bones. Carrying heavy shopping bags with handles looped around the fingers may induce body stress in the joints of the fingers or at the knuckles.

As a result, pain or stiffness will be experienced and possibly numbness or tingling. There may be weakness of the muscles when attempting to lift or grasp an object.

As the nerve supply to the arms and hands originates from the spinal nerves of the neck, it is essential that any body stress in the neck is released. In many instances, pain, stiffness and numbness in the arm or hand is due to compression in the neck and not to body stress in the arm itself.

The hip joint

The ball-shaped structure at the upper end of the thigh bone fits into a deep, secure socket in the pelvis. However, this joint may be stressed by movements such as mounting a bicycle or a horse, a fall, or from sitting cross-legged when unaccustomed to this position.

As tension becomes locked into the hip joint, mobility may become restricted, there may be a sharp, jabbing pain deep in the joint, or a milder ache when walking or dancing.

The knee joint

This joint undergoes a great deal of daily strain. Not only does it bear the weight of the body, but it is also designed to be a flexibile hinge joint. The cartilage pad in the knee joint and the ligaments supporting the joint may be stressed by twisting the knee, by jarring it in a fall, or in a hard kick.

When there is body stress in the knee, besides being painful the knee joint may be weakened to the point of collapsing when pressure is exerted on the leg, as in going up or down stairs.

The ankle and foot

Body stress may become locked into the joints if a person jars or twists an ankle, as in stepping off a pavement incorrectly, or in a kicking action. As well as pain, the ankle may collapse when the weight of the body is placed on that leg. The joints of the toes may also become stressed, and over time this may contribute to the development of a bunion.

As the nerve supply to the legs and feet originates from the spinal nerves of the lower back, it is vital that any body stress in this area of the spine is released. Very commonly, any pain, stiffness or numbness in the legs or feet is a result of compression in the lower back.

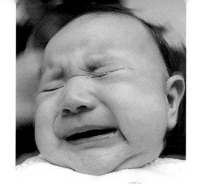

Babies may experience body stress, perhaps following a difficult birth.

BABIES AND CHILDREN

If the birth process was difficult, a baby may be born with body stress, especially in the neck and lower spine. A common sign that a baby has body stress in the neck is constant crying for no apparent reason. A baby with lower back body stress will cry when the hips are lifted during nappy changing. The

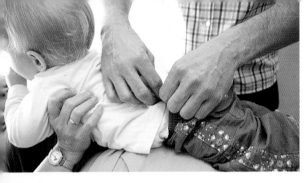

Under 18 months, a baby will be assessed for body stress with the BSR practitioner carrying out the tests while the baby lies on the mother's chest.

impact on the nervous system may cause constipation. Body stress in the area of the diaphragm may result in colic.

Small children are likely to accumulate body stress as a result of frequent falls and jerks while playing, or from trying to lift heavy objects.

Children may sit incorrectly. Reading or studying while sitting hunched over on a bed will induce stress in the neck and lower back. Watching television in a half-lying position, which reverses the normal lumbar curve, will cause pressure to build up in the spine.

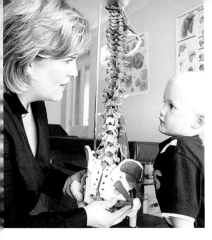
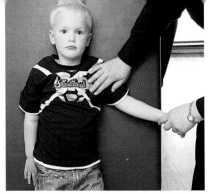

BSR can safely be carried out on toddlers and children.

As children approach puberty, they become more self-conscious and may develop poor posture. Hunched shoulders, a contracted chest, and a downward tilted head occur as a defensive mechanism against the new challenges and stresses of life. Muscles tighten and tension becomes locked into the body.

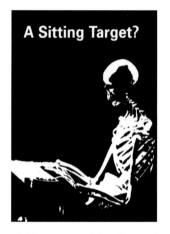

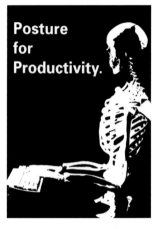

Children can avoid the effects of body stress accumulating by adopting good posture when studying, and by carrying bags in a backpack rather than slung over one shoulder.

Photos courtesy of Posturite.

Toddlers who refuse to walk and demand to be carried, or who complain of sore legs (so-called 'growing pains'), are likely to have body stress in the lower back. The leg muscles may be affected, causing a tendency to turn the feet inwards. Bed-wetting may occur if the nerve supply to the bladder is irritated.

THE HEALING POWER OF THE BODY

The body is an incredible creation, with an in-built ability for natural healing.

The brain co-ordinates healing via the nervous system, which, in turn, controls the function of every cell, tissue, organ and system of the body. It has controlling mechanisms that continuously adapt to both outside influences and to internal changes and stresses.

The body has two nervous systems:

- The Somatic Nervous System (SNS);
- The Autonomic Nervous System (ANS), which works automatically.

The Somatic Nervous System (SNS) includes all nerves controlling the muscular system and external sensory receptors.

The Autonomic Nervous System (ANS) is part of the peripheral nervous system and it controls the organs and involuntary muscles of the body. In most situations we are unaware of the workings of the ANS because it functions in an automatic, reflexive manner.

The Autonomic Nervous System is divided into:

- A sympathetic system: This is triggered by the 'fight or flight' reaction of an emergency and causes an increase in heart rate, rapid breathing, and decreased gastro-intestinal activity.
- A parasympathetic system: This causes a reduced heart rate and increased activity of the digestive system (for 'rest and digest').

The autonomic nervous system works continuously, not just during 'fight or flight' or 'rest and digest' situations. Its two systems work in harmony to maintain normal function.

*Body Stress Release has one objective only –
to enable the body to release its locked-in stress,
thereby allowing the body to restore the optimum
state of function. Freedom from body stress
promotes a better quality of life –
physically, mentally and emotionally.*

However, if stress becomes locked into an area of the body, the surrounding muscles tighten, compressing the nerves and thereby disturbing the body's ability to communicate. This impact on the nervous system undermines the body's functioning and its ability to heal itself.

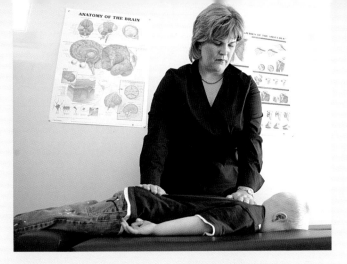

What Can Body Stress Release Help?

Body Stress Release is for all – from infants to the elderly. Clients coming for Body Stress Release are usually looking for relief from pain, stiffness or other discomfort.

While Body Stress Release is not a diagnosis nor a treatment for any specific condition or illness, it assists the body in restoring its self-healing capacity.

COMMON COMPLAINTS
Clients have reported improved health relating to a wide range of conditions, as follows.

Musculo-skeletal and neurological complaints

- *Back pain*
- *Sciatica*
- *'Slipped' discs*
- *Scoliosis*
- *Neck pain*
- *Arthritis*
- *Whiplash*
- *Hip pain*
- *Frozen shoulder*
- *Bad posture*
- *Repetitive Strain Injury*
- *Tennis elbow*
- *Migraines*
- *Headaches*
- *Dizziness*

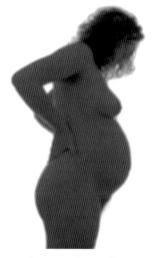

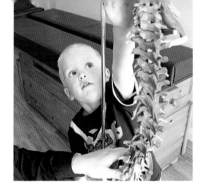

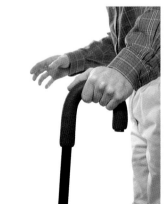

Body Stress release is for everyone, from infants to the elderly. It can also be safely carrried out during pregnancy. Clients coming for BSR are usually looking for relief from pain, stiffness and other discomfort.

- *Neuralgia*
- *Bell's palsy*
- *TMJ and grinding of teeth*

Respiratory conditions

- *Hay fever*
- *Asthma*
- *Recurring colds*
- *Sinusitis*
- *Catarrh*
- *Snoring*

Gastro-intestinal conditions

- *Heartburn*
- *Indigestion*
- *Irritable bowel syndrome*
- *Constipation*
- *Diarrhoea*

Emotional problems

- *Stress*
- *Insomnia*
- *Depression*
- *Anxiety*
- *Past trauma*
- *General fatigue*

Skin disorders:

- *Psoriasis*
- *Eczema*

Childhood conditions

- *Colic in babies*
- *Poor posture*
- *Bed-wetting (enuresis)*
- *Growing pains in children*

Wellness

- *Body Stress Release also has a broader objective. It is concerned with assisting 'wellness' and many people benefit from having regular releases to maintain health.*

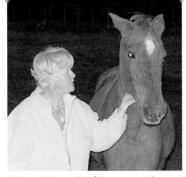

BSR can be used safely on animals, although not all practitioners attend to animals.

Animals

- *Body Stress Release can also safely be used on animals – including cats, dogs and horses – to enhance health. Animals often respond more quickly than humans and their owners exclaim in wonder at the results. N.B. Not all practitioners attend to animals.*

BSR COMPLEMENTS TRADITIONAL MEDICINE

Body Stress Release is not an alternative to allopathic or traditional medicine. It is complementary.

BSR practitioners have built good relationships with the medical world. GPs, orthopaedic surgeons, paediatricians, cardiologists and other specialists have referred patients for BSR. In many instances, surgery has been avoided.

Clients who are on medication are always advised to keep in close contact with their doctor. As BSR stimulates the body's self-healing power, the doctor may find that the dose needs to be reduced. This may apply to those with diabetes, high blood pressure, or asthma.

Referrals are made the other way, too. If a BSR practitioner notices that something is hindering the healing process or working against it, the client is advised to seek medical investigation and possibly screening. A client's mind can then be put at rest. If no underlying cause is found, often the symptoms may be attributed to locked-in body stress.

Clients undergoing BSR may find that, as the body starts to heal itself, the various medications they have been taking to suppress pain or discomfort (such as headaches or indigestion) may no longer be required.

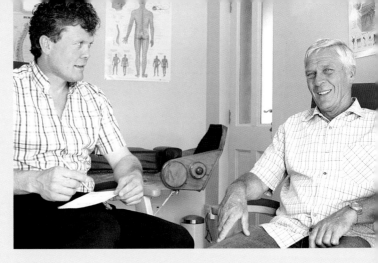

5

What Happens During
An Appointment?

Initially, a practitioner will recommend booking three appointments, which last approximately 30-45 minutes. Further appointments may be required, but as these are based on the individual's progress, the practitioner will advise.

CASE HISTORY

The practitioner takes a detailed case history and asks various questions about past operations, illnesses, fractures, accidents, emotional traumas, stress, type of exercise undertaken, specific aches and pains, and the reason for coming for Body Stress Release.

The practitioner gives an explanation of BSR and describes what will happen during the appointment.

'RELEASES'

Once the case history has been taken, the practitioner carries out the body stress tests and releases.

Some practitioners work on a portable couch, while others use a specially designed BSR 'hi-

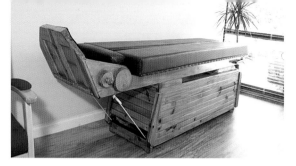

*The 'hi-lo'
BSR couch.*

lo' couch. This lowers the client from standing to a lying down position. Whichever table is used makes no difference to the quality of the releases.

Body Stress Release uses information provided by the body to determine where stored tension is undermining the efficiency of the nervous system and disturbing the body's ability to co-ordinate its functioning.

The practitioner locates body stress by using the body as a bio-feedback mechanism. Gentle pressure tests are conducted, working along the client's spine and other areas of the body.

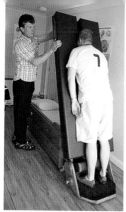
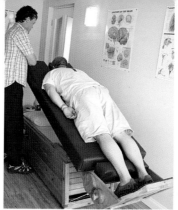

A client is lowered from standing to lying down on a 'hi-lo' BSR couch.

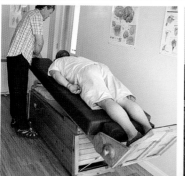
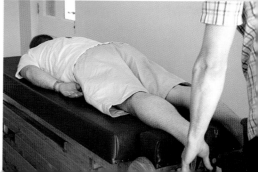

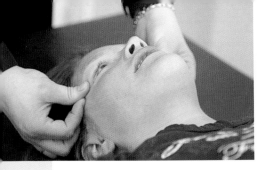
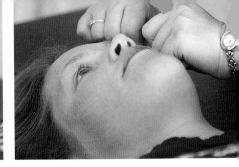

Carrying out 'releases'.

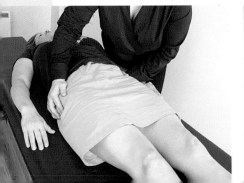
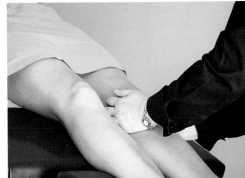

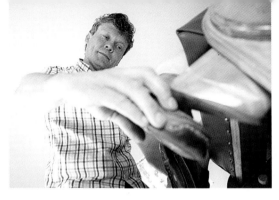

*'Reading
the monitor'*

The results of the tests are 'read' by the practitioner, observing the muscular responses while holding the client's feet. This is known in BSR terms as 'reading the monitor.'

Once the sites of body stress are located, the practitioner releases the tension by hand, using light but definite pressure. Certain areas may feel quite sensitive; however some people find the releases so relaxing that they fall asleep.

The body may let go of

49

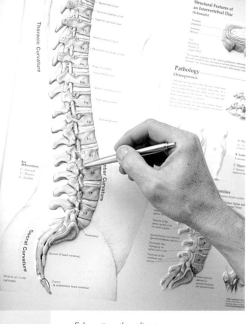

Educating the client.

locked-in tension rapidly but if stress has been stored for a long time, more releases may be required over a period of time. This is because the tight, protective layers of muscle tend to relax back to their normal tone in stages.

Clients are then provided with feedback on the findings. Simple self-help techniques are suggested and advice is given on the importance of good posture and correct exercising.

The cost of an appointment varies from £35-£60, depending on location.

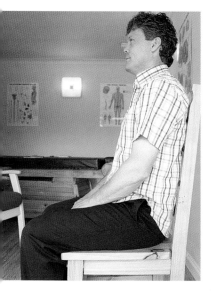 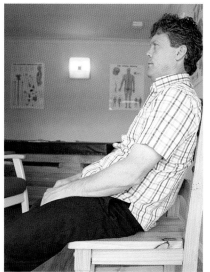

Demonstrating good and bad posture.

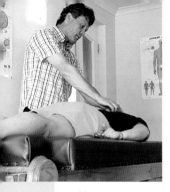 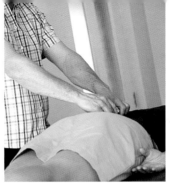 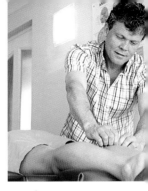

Maintenance appointments are recommended every two to three months.

MAINTENANCE APPOINTMENTS

After a client has completed the required BSR sessions, maintenance appointments every two to three months are recommended. In this way, any re-stressing of areas may be released before symptoms arise.

RETURNING SYMPTOMS

When a person has had a long-term condition of body stress, such as that originating from a past incident, there is an accumulation of layers of muscle tension. After several sessions of BSR there may be total relief from pain and other symptoms.

As time passes –possibly days, weeks or even months – the body will continue its process of unlocking a deeper level of stored tension. As the muscles relax back to their normal tone, there may be an uncovering of the original cause. A return of pain or stiffness means that the body is ready to deal with this with some further BSR sessions.

A client should not become despondent about a problem that seems to have returned. It is an indication that more stored tension needs to be attended to.

Body Stress Release is gentle, yet highly effective, and the body needs to be allowed time to respond to the releases. It is not advisable to undergo more than one type of complementary health technique at any one time, in the hope of a quick fix.

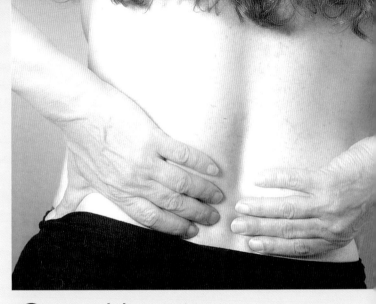

6

Case Histories

The following case histories illustrate how people with common complaints have benefited from the technique of Body Stress Release.

Jim, 49, came for BSR complaining of constant dizziness and pain in his right buttock since a fall down stairs, two years previously.

An MRI scan was clear. By the second appointment, Jim reported that the dizzy spells had gone, the pain in his buttock had completely disappeared, and he was feeling a lot better than he had done for years.

Margaret, 65, a carer for her physically disabled adult daughter, suffered lower back pain – the result of years of lifting – and depended on two sticks when walking. The pain was excruciating and made her weep on occasions. She also had rheumatoid arthritis in her fingers. She had been relying on medication prescribed by her GP to help with the pain.

When she read a newspaper article about BSR she decided, in

desperation, to try it. Even after the first few sessions she was less stooped and more upright.

Her back pain was less severe, she had reduced her use of painkillers, and now only required one stick when walking. In addition, her fingers were no longer swollen and had miraculously straightened.

Philippa, a 48-year-old therapist, had been experiencing pain in her neck and left shoulder, as well as having problems with a weak left wrist, since being knocked over by a car three months previously. She also suffered back pain on her right side.

Just two appointments improved the situation considerably, with the client reporting that there was no longer any pain in her shoulder, neck or lower back.

Ginny, 69, first had Body Stress Release in South Africa, after being 'crippled' from hours spent in a car during an arduous driving holiday.

Having had a bad back and arthritis for years, she had more

or less come to accept her problems as an inevitable part of the ageing process.

After only one release she was amazed with the results, and continued with a further course on her return to the UK. She described the feeling of BSR as though it had 'unravelled' the muscle aches and pains she had experienced for years. She now attends maintenance releases every couple of months as she finds it beneficial.

Harry, 4, came for BSR following a tobogganing accident.

Hospital X-rays showed no broken bones but internal bleeding in the leg, which the doctors had advised would heal in a couple of weeks.

At his first appointment Harry was unable to bear weight on the leg and was experiencing pain. Releases were carried out and his mother reported that Harry was running around, obviously free from pain, within four days. By the second appointment, a week later, he came in without his leg brace and reported that the leg was 'much better, thank you!'

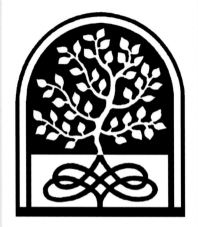

UNLOCKING TENSION –
RESTORING SELF-HEALING

The BSR logo

7

Resources

The Body Stress Release Association (UK) is affiliated to The Body Stress Release Association in South Africa.

Practitioners who successfully complete the intensive, full-time five-month training course with theoretical and practical examinations in South Africa and who intend to practise in the UK are required to join the UK Association Practitioners are covered by professional indemnity insurance and are involved in continuing professional development.

The Body Stress Release Association (UK) is a full-member organisation of the British Complementary Medicine Association (www.bcma.co.uk)

To find a practitioner, contact:
Body Stress Release Association (UK):
www.bodystressrelease-uk.co.uk
Body Stress Release International:
www.bodystressrelease.com

To find out about training, contact:
Paul Masureik
Tel: +44 (0)1276 475 651
Email: paul@bodystressrelease.co.uk
Postal Address:
The Body Stress Release
Association (UK),
Shrublands Drive,
Lightwater,
Surrey GU18 5QS.

GLOSSARY OF BSR TERMINOLOGY

BSR has its own specific terminology that practitioners use. The following terminology is provided as a means of reference to assist understanding.

Assessment: The procedure followed to establish the presence of stress patterns.

Appointment/Release/Session/Visit: A BSR practitioner will use these words interchangeably. The word treatment is never used. In BSR, practitioners do not treat or diagnose any specific condition or illness.

Adaptation: A term used to describe re-tightening of superficial muscles.

Body stress: The presence of tension stored within the body.

Body Stress Release: A health profession, not a healing profession.

Centre/Office/Practice/Rooms: These term may be used interchangeably. The words clinic or surgery will not be used.

Client: The person coming for BSR. The word patient is never used.

Complementary Health Profession/Complementary Health Technique or Modality: A generic term used to describe the practise of BSR.

Health: A condition of optimal function – physically, mentally and emotionally.

Healing: The natural ability of the body to restore itself to health. It is not carried out by an outside influence, although the body may be assisted or stimulated in its healing process by an outside influence, which may be regarded as a catalyst.

Monitor: The body's response mechanism to the stress tests carried out on the client by the practitioner.

Lines of tension/compression/pressure: Terminology used by a BSR practitioner to refer to sites of body stress, which may be undermining the body's ability to function at optimum level. This term should not be confused with pressure points.

Release/s: The procedure applied to areas of body stress, carried out by the BSR practitioner on the client.

Stress: As a noun this refers to cause – i.e. chemical, mechanical or emotional. As a verb it refers to stress in an area of the body.

About the author

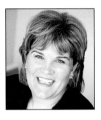

Kerry Teakle was Scotland's first Body Stress Release practitioner and had held the position of Chairperson of the Body Stress Release Association (UK). She is also a Bach Foundation Registered Practitioner (BFRP) and a freelance public relations consultant, working for a variety of clients.

Kerry is a Board Trustee and Affiliate Professional Member of BackCare, advising on their PR and marketing. BackCare is an independent national charity committed to reducing the impact of back pain.
www.backcare.org.uk

Chronic back pain led Kerry to retrain in BSR in South Africa in 2003, under Gail and Ewald Meggersee. She has also completed the intensive review and advanced workshop at the BSR Academy in 2005. Kerry practises at Medicalternative, a private GP practice, in Edinburgh. For appointments contact:
0131 225 5656/0780 110 3528
www.medicalternative.com

ACKNOWLEDGEMENTS
Thanks are due to: Gail and Ewald Meggersee for the use of copyrighted material; the BSRA Board of Trustees (SA); The Body Stress Release Association (UK); Ian Soutar for use of his BSR practice in Letham, Angus for the photographic shoot; the Gilroy family and Dave Soutar who modelled for the photographs; Backcare and Posturite for use of some images; and Ally Stuart Photography.